Dina & Brad —

Here's to worrying less & living very long.
Bijal's a good friend — Enjoy. With love
Maika

The Breathing Breakthrough

Also by Bija Bennett

Emotional Yoga:
How the Body Can Heal the Mind

Breathing into Life:
Recovering Wholeness Through Body,
Mind & Breath

The Workout:
Feeling Great Again — Strength

Stress Reduction:
Feeling at Home — Relaxation

Finding Focus:
Feeling Clarity of Mind — Concentration

A Good Night from YogaAway

The Breathing Breakthrough

Everything You Need to Know to Sharpen Your Focus, Worry Less, and Live Longer

Bija Bennett

Copyright © 2016 Bija Bennett, Inc.

All rights reserved. No part of this book may be used or reproduced by any means, graphic, electronic, or mechanical, including photocopying, recording, taping or by any information storage retrieval system without the written permission of the author except in the case of brief quotations embodied in critical articles and reviews.

Balboa Press books may be ordered through booksellers or by contacting:

Balboa Press
A Division of Hay House
1663 Liberty Drive
Bloomington, IN 47403
www.balboapress.com
1 (877) 407-4847

Because of the dynamic nature of the Internet, any web addresses or links contained in this book may have changed since publication and may no longer be valid. The views expressed in this work are solely those of the author and do not necessarily reflect the views of the publisher, and the publisher hereby disclaims any responsibility for them.

Black and White Photographs: Lois Greenfield
Author Photograph: Todd Rosenberg
Other Photographs: Bija Bennett Films

ISBN: 978-1-5043-4368-8 (sc)
ISBN: 978-1-5043-4369-5 (e)

Print information available on the last page.

Balboa Press rev. date: 1/20/2016

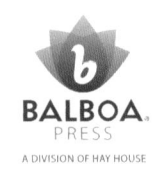

Contents

The Breathing Breakthrough   1
Risking Stress   1
Evidence-Based Practices   3
The facts   3
The solution   3
Ancient Science, Modern Results   4
The sciences of Panchamaya   5
This is the Art of Yoga   5
The Breathing Breakthrough   6
Breathing as Stress Reduction Therapy   6

Breathing Lessons   7
The Basic Components of Breathing   7
Guidelines for Breathing   8
Strategic Breathing:
Five Practices for Life   10
Practice 1: Breathing Awareness   10
Practice 2: The Whispering Breath   10
Practice 3: The Wave   11
Practice 4: Balancing Breath   12
*Practice 5: Reducing and
Nourishing Breaths*   12

**Breathing Rituals:
For Body-Mind Recovery**   14
Your Body and Your Breath   14
Your Mind and Your Breath   16
Your Emotions and Your Breath   17
Your Immunity and Your Breath   18
Breathing into Life   19

The Breathing Breakthrough

You probably think you already know how to breathe. Isn't breathing one of those things that, under normal circumstances, you never have to think about, like hearing or seeing? Yes, but it shouldn't be. You can go through your whole life and never give your breathing another thought, and that's why it might never occur to you that you're not breathing maximally or getting the most out of your breath.

Did you know that your breathing can release stress, maximize energy, strengthen immunity, increase circulation, improve digestion, align posture, promote relaxation, help you focus, reduce pain and fear, and therefore, lead to a longer and healthier life?

The breath is remarkable. You can learn a lot from the breath. It is profoundly wise.

Every emotion, physical condition, resistance, disturbance, or tension you have is connected to your breath. Do you ever notice that you're holding your breath? Remember what you do when you're afraid, tense, or worrying about something? Or how you breathe when you feel happy? Or sad? Or when you've been sitting at your desk all day?

Your breathing always carries a message. Your breath can be your best friend. It can be a tool to balance, release and free your mind and body. It can bring you strength and courage. It can calm you down. It can give you energy. It can even lessen obsessive-compulsive, anxious, and attention-deficit states — which break you down — merely by letting some air rush in.

Breathing is an art. But you don't need to be taught how to breathe to survive. You already know how to do that. *Now it's time for your breathing to be liberated!*

Risking Stress

We live in an age of terrifying speed and haste. Everything we do is at high speed. We even gobble our food down quickly. We've created all sorts of quick devices that let us save another fraction of a second. 'Time is money' has become 'speed is money.' But speed has consequences. And, racing around rarely allows us to pause and consider what we're doing, where we want to go, and how we want to be when we get there.

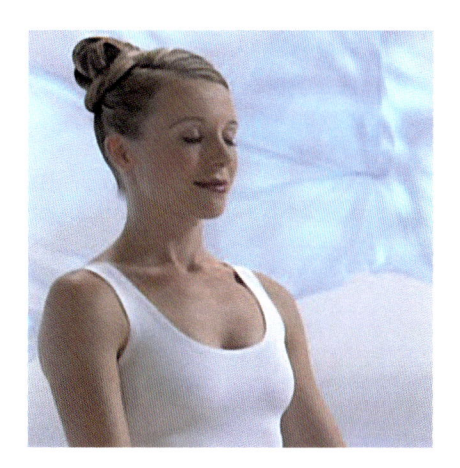

'The breath is remarkable. You can learn a lot from the breath. It is profoundly wise'

From the moment we wake up we have deadlines, frustrations, and demands. We're pushed to engage, produce, and perform. Even managing our time isn't much of a relief. Faced with an already overburdened state, we still need the energy it takes to stay mentally focused, physically energized, and emotionally connected.

What's really driving us mad is our continuous plugged-in state. While technology changes everything, it's dangerous and delusional to deny that our all-pervasive obsession with continuously being connected to our computer devices and cell phones isn't making us more anxious, stressed-out, depressed, sleep-deprived and maybe even a little less self-aware.

The proof is starting to pile up. In his July, 2012 *Newsweek* article, Tony Dokoupil, reported the hard facts:

- Internet addiction physically alters our brains, in the areas of attention, control and primary function.

- Americans stare at a computer screen for an average of eight hours a day. And teenagers stare at a screen, including time on iPhones, iPads, etc., around eleven hours each day.

- More than one-third of smart phone users get online before getting out of bed.

- An astounding six-figure number of texts per month we get are typical.

'We're wired up, but we're melting down'

Tony Schwartz

One in ten smart phone users consider themselves 'addicted' to their phones. Studies show that people, often students, are 'not just unwilling, but are functionally unable to be without their media links to the world.' And, with the exception of those 50 and over, many individuals check text messages, email or their social network, 'all the time' or every 15 minutes, a pathology we consider normal.

This correlates to performance in the workplace, as multi-tasking, 'cognitive overload,' and the accompanying effect of reduced efficiency, forgetfulness, work errors, lost business, and sick time, all directly affect the bottom line.

A study from The Energy Project, founded by author and performance expert Tony Schwartz, continues to demonstrate the data. In a 2008 Towers Perin Global Workforce Study of 90,000 employees across 18 countries, only 20% of them, one out of every five, felt 'fully engaged' at work. In other words, over 40% were actively 'dis-engaged.'

The data suggests that the challenges of stress, engagement, and recovery are the same for all corporate cultures, and that it doesn't matter who you are and where you are from, the constant urgency and endless distractions are undermining our ability to perform at our best.

As it turns out, 'we're wired up but we're melting down,' says Schwartz. And it's not getting any better faster.

Then, of course, we have habits that include continuous late night working, not getting enough sleep, drinking too much, and not eating when we're hungry, which override our ability to recover. The result is a combination of weight gain, sleep deprivation, high blood pressure, a decrease in brain function — all health markers related to the lack of recovery, which, on a chronic basis, creates dire consequences.

This is a serious problem because it means that at some point we've probably damaged our metabolism. Damage occurs by creating more stress in the system than it can handle. It happens when we allow our habits to physiologically break us down, and when we let our nutrition, sleep, and lifestyle habits interrupt our ability to recuperate. When symptoms increase and we're more tired, stressed out, not as happy, or aging faster than it seems we have before, it's time to make significant changes.

Extreme as it may seem, unless we pay attention to the degree of stress we take in vs. the degree to which we rebuild, recover, and repair, we are killing ourselves even faster. In truth, 'our attention is under siege,' and now more than ever, we need a full-blown recovery system with highly specific routines that help us reduce stress and manage our energy at every level.

Depending on the quality of our lifestyle habits and choices, the good news is we can rebuild our metabolism and improve our health right now. But no matter what, says metabolism expert and endocrinologist Diana Schwarzbein, M.D., 'You have to find ways to manage your stress, or you can never be fully healthy.'

Evidence-Based Practices

The facts
Stress, in whatever form it takes, can trigger the release of powerful hormones, which flood the brain engaging the 'fight or flight' response — changes your body goes through in response to stress. These changes may manifest as increased heart rate, narrowing of vision, muscle tension, and sweating. Common acute stress symptoms also include: headaches, insomnia, hyperactivity, fatigue, digestive issues, nervousness, anxiety, overeating, loss of enthusiasm, mood changes, irritability, depression — to name a few.

'You have to find ways to manage your stress, or you can never be fully healthy'
Diana Schwarzbein, M.D.

The solution
Balancing stress and recovering from it is critical to managing your energy in all facets of your life. When you recover your energy, you nourish your system and fill it back up. Without it, you burn yourself out and eventually break down. But stress itself is not the enemy. It's a stimulus that helps you to use up your energy and then recover from it, so you get stronger and stronger.

Growing, in every part of your life, requires you to skillfully manage both of these parts — the expending as well as the recovering. Over time, this is what sustains your life and supports your growth. And it's a discipline you must launch for yourself.

Ultimately, stress is personal. When facing the truth in dealing with your stress and the ability to respond to your stress, you're going to have to deal with the most fundamental relationship you have — the relationship you have with yourself. And what's more intimate to yourself than your breath?

If you could feel more positive and mentally focused, have more fun, and renew your energy so that you could engage positively in every area of your life, including relationships and work, simply by harnessing the power of your breath, wouldn't you?

Evidence-based research strongly shows that by adding mind-body and self-care techniques, you can significantly create an impact on a diverse range of health responses — from energy, aging, brain and immune strength, to sleep, happiness, family, intimacy, and even sex.

New clinical trials on stress reduction demonstrate that people who adopt yoga-based, breathing-centered therapies considerably reduce their perceived stress levels and improve their ability to respond to stress in a big way. This includes improved quality of sleep, decreased anxiety and depression, regulation of pain responses, reduced blood levels of stress hormones, improved cardiovascular function, and increased brain wave synchrony.

The Harvard Mental Health Letter also reports encouraging results for people practicing yoga and breathing. Indicators include: modulating stress response systems, toning down maladaptive nervous system arousal (as with post-traumatic stress disorder), and increasing the central nervous system's ability to recover and rejuvenate in para- sympathetic mode, reducing your 'fight or flight' response.

Early adaptors in the health care industry are taking this seriously by identifying self-care as a value. The Aetna Group, in collaboration with Duke Integrative Medicine, eMindful and the American Viniyoga Institute, has decided to take a proactive approach to the health of their corporate culture. Recently, Aetna completed a clinical trial using their own employees, looking at mind-body stress reduction programs and other variables in the workplace.

They found that using therapeutic Viniyoga practices — movements, breathing techniques, guided relaxation, and mental skills — helped by reducing perceived stress in participants by 33 percent. Published in the *Journal of Occupational Health Psychology*, the study has led to an increasing adoption of wellness practices that reduce the burden of stress-related disease.

Says Aetna Chairman and CEO Mark T. Bertolini, 'Stress can have a significant impact on physical and mental health. The results from the mind-body study, provides evidence that these mind-body approaches can be an effective complement to conventional medicine and may help people improve their health, something that I have experienced personally.'

Aetna's approach includes a rigorous sequence of lifestyle rituals for the body, mind, and emotions, as well as relational and spiritual attitudes and behaviors — all essential keys for creating optimal health. Eating regularly, sleeping enough, exercising the body, resting and recovering, making boundaries between home and work, along with meditation skills and breathing techniques are options and choices that recalibrate energy, enhance a healthy metabolism and build the foundation for a passionate and satisfying life. It's time to build important personal energy management strategies for life.

Ancient Science, Modern Results

Where did the strategies for self-care come from? Some are new, some are old, and some are ancient even, dating back to ninth-century India.

Long before science validated the connection between the body and the brain, the ancient Indian masters understood how one part of our system influenced all other parts, and that our body, mind, and emotions are a part of one integrated system, and when we influence one aspect of our system we affect every other aspect.

They knew that we are the sum of a broad range of complexities and, consequently, created a series of complete sciences or integrative therapies for refining and developing each aspect of who we are. Called *Panchamaya*, or five layers, this model of wellness compiles an extraordinary library of knowledge about the body and mind.

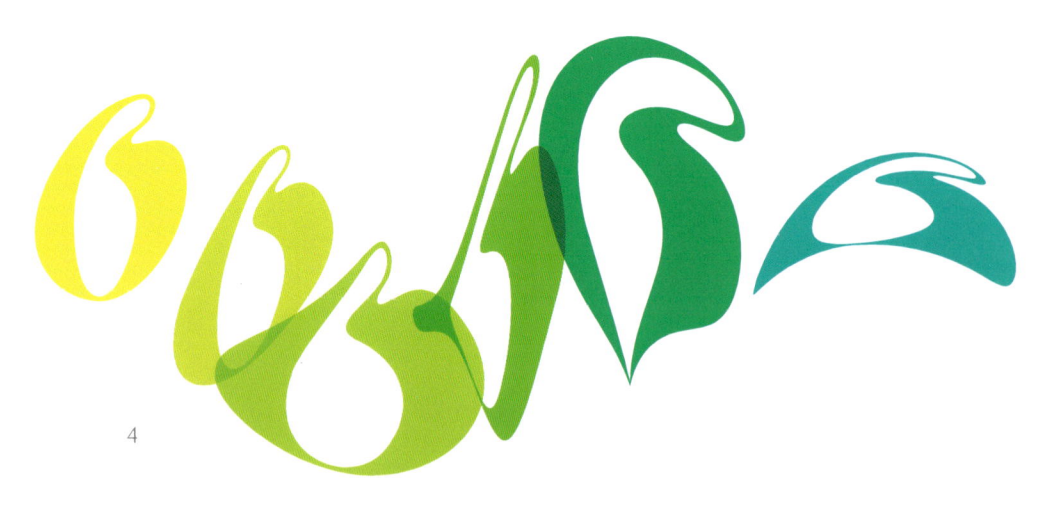

The sciences of *Panchamaya*

For physical strength and flexibility, the ancient masters created the disciplines of *asana*, or conscious movement.

For the physiology, they created the practice of *pranayama*, or conscious breathing.

Chanting was used to support the mind.

For the development of behavior and human character they articulated the science of *meditation*.

Ritual and prayer brought it all together as a personal practice.

Still relevant to us today, these sciences deliberately deal with our everyday issues — anxiety, stress, depression, and fear. Each one unfolds a particular technique or tool to transform and heal our lives at each level.

This is the Art of Yoga

Yoga, as it was initially designed, is one of the oldest forms of self-care in the world. Unfortunately, yoga in our present culture is generally misunderstood.

'Each time you attempt to link with any aspect of yourself or your world, you are doing yoga'

The basic Western misunderstanding of yoga is that it's merely separate positions to be mastered. *It is not.* Yoga is not just physical training, positions or movements — it is not even primarily about exercise. *Yoga is an ancient, practical system for accessing, healing, and integrating the body and mind.*

Yoga practices involve our feelings, our thoughts, and our emotional flexibility. In yoga, it doesn't really matter if your hamstring muscles are tight. Yoga is much more a state of mind than having to touch your toes.

The word *yoga* comes from the Sanskrit word *yuj*, which means to 'join, link, or connect.' The essence of yoga is yoking or uniting, and to practice yoga is to 'join with' — to reach a new level of integration within yourself. Yoga is the art of linking to all parts of yourself — your body, your thoughts, your awareness, your emotions, and your breath.

Each time you attempt to link with any aspect of yourself or your world, you are doing yoga.

In yoga, conscious breathing is called *pranayama*. According to the yogic texts, breathing is the vehicle that carries the life force, or *prana*, throughout your body.

But *prana* is more than breathing. *Prana* is life. It is vibratory power. *Prana* connects your body to your mind and to your consciousness and spirit. Through *prana*, you not only feel alive, but you're able to extend your life force to others, and to guide your energy, thoughts, and desires.

As you regulate the flow of *prana*, or breath, in your body, you affect the quality of your mind. When breathing slows down, your thinking process slows, and you attain steadiness. When your mind becomes still, breathing is calm. When your breathing almost stops, your mind comes to a standstill and you enter a state of 'restful alertness.' This is the beginning of meditation.

The science of *pranayama*, or conscious breathing, uses the breath as a vehicle for healing and balance. Considered the primary tool for self-development in yoga, *pranayama* helps you to contact deeper and subtler physical, mental, and emotional states by making conscious what is ordinarily an unconscious pattern of breathing. Creating a state of restful alertness, *pranayama* promotes lucidity and mental clarity. It calms agitated states, such as anger and anxiety, and improves the vitality of your body and mind.

The Breathing Breakthrough

The Breathing Breakthrough teaches you how to link your awareness with your breath to create optimal health. 'Conscious awareness' is a mystical sounding term that simply refers to an awareness of everything about you, including your body, your mind, and your breath.

It means that you *actively participate with your breath* and choose to consciously feel your physical and emotional responses. This provides you with the 'medicine of awareness,' the real medicine your body and mind especially need.

Breathing as Stress Reduction Therapy

Research into the respiratory process confirms that the quality of your breathing has dramatic physical effects on both your body and mind. Through slow, conscious, rhythmic respiration, using the movement of your diaphragm, you can increase your relaxation response; decrease your metabolic rate and blood-sugar levels; lower your heart rate; reduce muscle tension, fatigue, and pain; and increase strength, mental and physical alertness, confidence, and emotional stability. Pretty good for just some breathing!

Breathing balances your mind and brings concentration, mental vitality, and the ability to discern more clearly how your thoughts and emotions often distort your perception. Breathing thus reveals the essence of an emotion.

Breathing is also a mirror of your body and mind's reactions. It acts as a kind of safety valve: If you're overstressed, your breathing is irregular and short; if you're happy, your breathing is steady and long. By observing your breathing, you can be alert to what's happening within your body and mind. Once you're familiar with your breath's many variations and modulations, and how they affect you, you can balance how you feel at any time and in any situation.

Directing your attention to the process of breathing becomes a powerful tool to optimize health, increase longevity, dissolve fear, manage your emotions and develop higher states of consciousness. It's simply the easiest and most powerful stress reduction tool you can use to support, manage, and sustain your health regardless of your age or condition.

> 'Research into the respiratory process confirms that the quality of your breathing has dramatic physical effects on both your body and mind'

Breathing Lessons

Remember, this is not a breathing class. This is your breath, *and this is your life*. No one is going to judge you, test you, or give you a grade.

So, let's get honest about where your breath is right now. Do you feel yourself straining as you inhale? Notice any resistance. And take your time. Allow your exhale to become a little longer and slower. Don't let the out-breath release too fast. Notice if you collapse your body as you breathe out. Instead, feel a slight contraction of your belly as you exhale slowly. Let your breathing become smooth and easy. *And just keep watching your breath.*

You can keep your eyes open and even continue reading as you breathe in and out easily and effortlessly. *Stay with your breath* for a moment. You can even close your eyes and just be with yourself and your breath. It's okay to put this page down so you can try this.

Give your breath some freedom again. Feel what's going on inside you right now. Notice your thoughts. Notice your feelings. Stay with your breath. And let the flow of your breath lead you to your present state of energy and awareness.

There is nothing you need to do. Just allow your awareness to be with your breath. Listen. And respect yourself. Then you will see that everything you are looking for is *right there.*

The Basic Components of Breathing

The simplest definition of yogic breathing, or *pranayama*, is 'to be with the breath.' What makes the practices of *pranayama* unique is that your attention is on the breath rather than on your body. This happens when you deliberately control your breathing cycle by regulating one or more of your breath's four parts:

1. Exhalation
2. Hold or retention with empty lungs
3. Inhalation
4. Hold or retention with full lungs

The pause, marking the point at which the collapse of the breath occurs, is called *kumbhaka* ('pot') in Sanskrit. This pause naturally comes after each incoming and each outgoing breath.

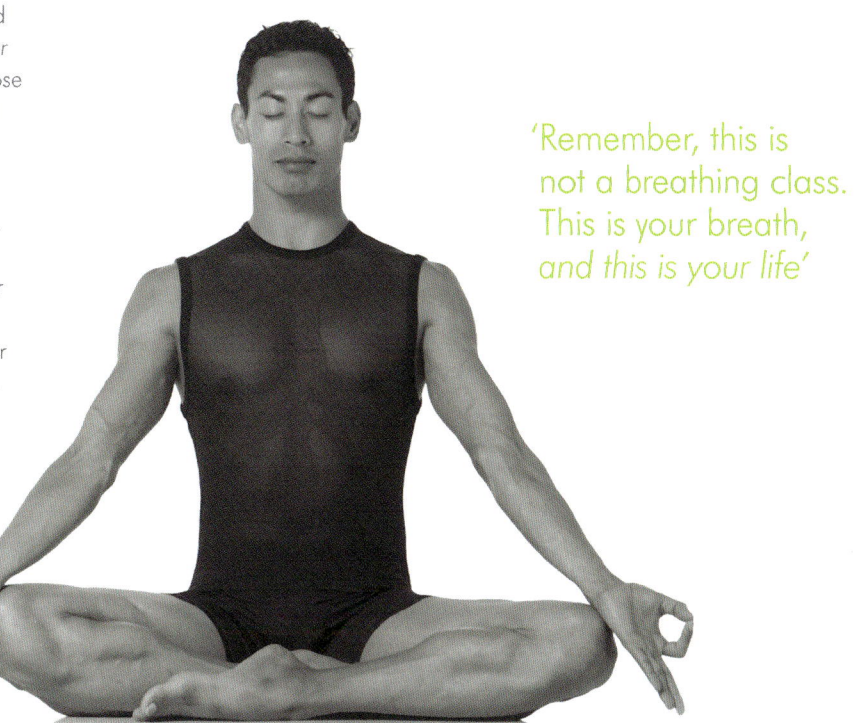

'Remember, this is not a breathing class. This is your breath, *and this is your life*'

'The Breathing Breakthrough teaches you how to link your awareness with your breath to create optimal health'

All yogic breathing exercises are created from modifying one or more of these four phases of breath and combining them in relation to one another. It's that simple. Yet, not always so easy. The point is to learn how to use your breath intelligently and be conscious of how and why you breathe.

Guidelines for Breathing

Here are a few important guidelines to conscious breathing:

1. When you begin the practice of breathing, you must follow a certain order. First, learn the components of the breath. Then, explore the biology of breathing. You will get the hang of it in no time.

2. Begin the practice of breathing according to your ability, concentrating on exhalation, inhalation, and retention, in that order.

    You can then work toward lengthening each phase.

    Never hold your breath, and never inhale or exhale with force. Be especially careful when holding your breath after inhalation, since pressure may build up in the muscles. Increase the length of your breathing gradually.

    If you feel any strain in your eyes, head, mouth, neck, shoulders, or spine, ease off and rest.

    Keep your hands relaxed and your mouth soft. Start with shorter breathing cycles and gradually work toward lengthening them. Advance slowly.

3. Practice breathing while sitting straight, in a comfortable position, with your eyes closed.

    Many breathing exercises can be practiced seated or lying down. Choosing one or the other changes the way you experience the exercise. Sitting supports more alertness. Lying down tends to relax you or even put you to sleep. Find the best posture by asking your body what it wants to do. There is no one correct position for breathing, except when practicing certain more complex techniques. The longer you practice, the easier the position you'll need.

    It's important to cultivate good posture for breathing. The truth is, breathing actually helps you to improve your posture. When you're breathing in a prone position, try lying down on a mat or blanket, or lying on the floor with pillows under your knees and head. Try a supported seated position on a couch or chair, or sitting on the floor with or without a blanket or pillow for support. Try them all. Be flexible. Sustain a good, seated position for some time and stay comfortable, and you will unite your body and mind and start floating in the present moment.

    If you're reading this in an airport, or on an airplane, or at your desk, you are already in a seated position. I find that airplanes are one of the best places to practice breathing. When I'm flying, I put my earphones on so nobody bothers me. Your desk is a great place, too. Even as I write this, I can take my hands off the keyboard, close my eyes, and breathe for a moment. It's like recess.

4 Keeping your mouth closed, breathe with a smooth and subtle sound passing from your throat through your nostrils.

Close your mouth and breathe through your nose. Deliberately begin The Whispering Breath from the back of your throat. (See Practice 2 — The Whispering Breath.) If some phlegm develops in your throat as you breathe, don't worry, that's normal. Simply take a little bit of warm water and gargle first to help clear your throat for breathing. You can also use The Whispering Breath when you work out.

5 Only when your breath is smooth and long should you progress to altering your breath's various components.

It takes a little practice to make your breath smooth and long. It's worth taking the time, though. If you don't, you'll miss something valuable. Slow down and notice what you didn't notice. Then you can begin to monitor your breath's other components:

- **Time and ratio** is the length, or duration of your inhalation, exhalation, and retention, which creates an equal or unequal ratio of breathing.

- **Number of breaths** is how many times you repeat a certain ratio, or component, of the breath. For example, inhaling for six counts, exhaling for six, then repeating this cycle four times.

- **Building a ratio or breathing threshold** is a strategy that takes you step by step, progressively preparing your breath for the main goal, and then gradually bringing you out of it.

- **The focus of your attention** often follows your breath as it comes into your chest area. On exhalation, your attention is naturally drawn to your belly.

- **The quality of your breath** should be long, slow, and refined, not too loud, and never rough. Use the sound of your breath to monitor any difficulty with your practice. Pay attention, and ask yourself: What is the sound of my breath? Is it steady and smooth? Loud or quiet? What is the duration? Is it short or long? Am I aware of the pauses between my breaths? What's going on in my mind as I breathe? Is my posture comfortable? Do I feel hot or cold? Notice the way your body responds during and after your practice.

- **Resting.** If you have time, lie down and rest at the end of your breathing practice. Stay a little while without getting up, and make a gradual transition into your next activity. Do this, and you'll feel better. If you feel tension building in your neck and shoulders, in your upper back, between your shoulder blades, in your jaw, or around your eyes, or if you feel more irritated than when you began, you're probably going beyond what's comfortable for you. Stop, lie down, and feel where the tension is. Then go back and find the natural ease with which your breath moves. If this tension happens regularly, check with a qualified teacher.

'Guidelines for Breathing' is an excerpt from *Emotional Yoga: How the Body Can Heal the Mind* (Simon and Schuster, 2002)

> 'Pay attention, and ask yourself: What is the sound of my breath? Is it steady and smooth? Loud or quiet? What is the duration? Is it long or short? What is going on in my mind as I breathe?'

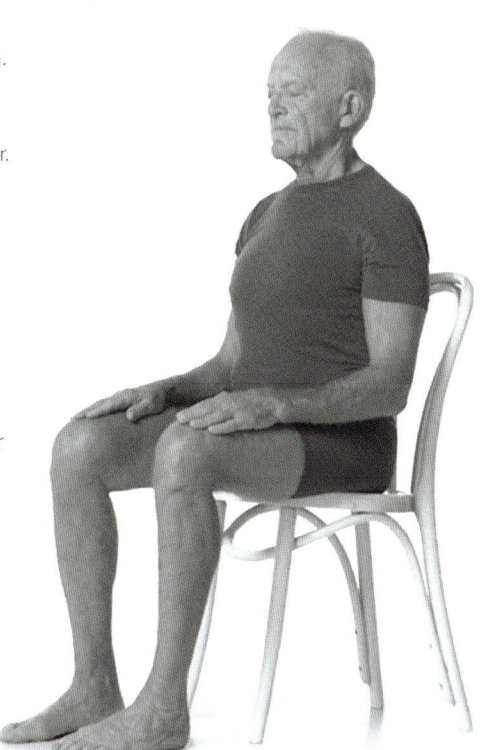

Strategic Breathing: Five Practices for Life

Breathing is one of the greatest secrets of yoga. If you practice it with sincerity, you will obtain healing powers beyond your imagination. Yet, breathing itself is not a secret. It's right there. If you train yourself in one area only, *be awake to your breath*. It's that basic. You can build your whole life around it.

Practice 1: Breathing Awareness

Effects: Settles and soothes your agitated emotional states, such as anger, anxiety, frustration, and fear. Relaxes your body. Calms your mind. Creates a state of 'restful alertness.'

- Sit comfortably, and shift your attention to the flow of your breath. Observe how it comes and goes. Ride your breath like a wave. Inhale and pause. Then exhale and pause. Inhale all the way to the end of your breath and feel the completion of your breath, waiting for your next breath to begin.

Exhale all the way to the end, and feel the completion of your breath, waiting for your next breath to begin. Lengthen your breath naturally, following it with awareness.

- Notice that as your physical breath ends, a part of it continues on an energetic level. Feel it come to its completion in silence. Wait in that silence. With every new breath, allow your attention to rest more deeply into the pause. Feel how your breath begins as an energetic pulse, then moves into your physical body and takes you with it into your next inhaling breath.

- Your breath comes in, and stops. Your breath goes out, and stops. It's effortless. You are pouring the inward into the outward breath, and the outward into the inward breath. Then, your breath ceases flowing in the silent space between each breath. Listen to the silence. Surrender to it, and breathe again. *Be in that silence*. Feel yourself turning back upon yourself as you breathe.

Practice 2: The Whispering Breath

Effects: Helps control and deepen the flow of your breath. Brings your attention inside. Focuses your awareness. Relaxes your body. Calms your mind.

- If you're not already breathing with a soft airy sound, try this. Whisper the word '*Ha*' and listen to where this breath originates in your throat.

Now, close your mouth, breathe through your nose, and create this same soft whispering sound when you breathe from the back of your throat without vocalizing. It sounds smooth and light, a rushing sound, like the wind through the trees. Keep this air sound going softly, both on your inhalation and exhalation.

- You are consciously controlling the flow of your breath by creating a valve as you slightly contract the glottis muscle at the back of your throat. Feel the sensation of the breath in your throat rather than in your nose. Breathe slowly and deeply, and listen to the sound of your breath. Let the air do it for you. There is no need to force it in or out. Just keep your breathing very smooth. And feel the sensation. I call this The Whispering Breath.

- This breathing technique is known as *Ujjayi Pranayama*. It helps you to stay focused and attentive; invigorates as well as calms your body and allows you to extend, lengthen, and deepen your breathing during almost anything you do — working out, walking, running, or simply sitting as a breathing practice. The more strongly you do it, the more of a heating effect it has. The slower and softer you do it, the more of a cooling effect it has.

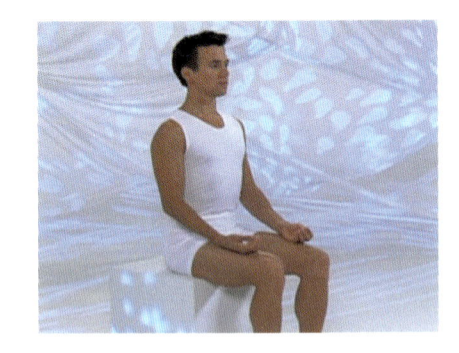

'Breathing is simply the easiest and most powerful stress reduction tool you can use to support, manage, and sustain your health'

Practice 3: The Wave

Effects: Encourages the movement of your diaphragm, massaging your organs, heart and lungs; facilitates the movement of your spine; improves your posture, respiration, digestion, elimination.

- On your next inhalation, begin to emphasize the action in your upper chest first, allowing your breath to move down toward your navel. Inhalation from your chest, rather than your belly, encourages the expansion of your rib cage, the lengthening and extension of your spine, and the stretching of the front of your body.

- When you inhale, your diaphragm contracts downward, allowing the air to be drawn into your lungs. Inhaling from your chest rather than from your belly facilitates the extension of your spine, the elevation of your rib cage, and the expansion of your chest.

- As you exhale, progressively tighten your abdominal muscles from the pubic bone (a few inches below your navel) to your belly, and from your belly to your solar plexus (gut). You will feel a slight gathering motion back into the center of your belly as your lower back rounds. Exhalation encourages your abdomen to contract and your lower spine to stretch.

- NOTE: This is NOT 'belly breathing,' which starts by filling the belly first on inhale and progressively filling the lungs from the bottom up.

- While this technique may seem counter-intuitive, try it, and eventually it will become easy.

- When you exhale, your diaphragm moves upward, pushing the air up and out. As you consciously contract your belly on exhale, you stabilize the connection between your pelvis and your lower back. This is good for you, and supports your lower back.

- Inhalation is a wave from the top down, and exhalation is a wave from the bottom up. The inhale moves in and down. The exhale moves up and out. As your diaphragm moves, your breath moves, and as your breath moves, your spine moves. (This too, helps your posture).

- Continue breathing in this wavelike motion, and keep your attention on the natural rhythmic flow of your breath. Through this smooth, gradual, even flow, your body is released back into its natural motion. I call this The Wave. It's a magnificent motion of your breath.

'The Wave. It's a magnificent motion of your breath'

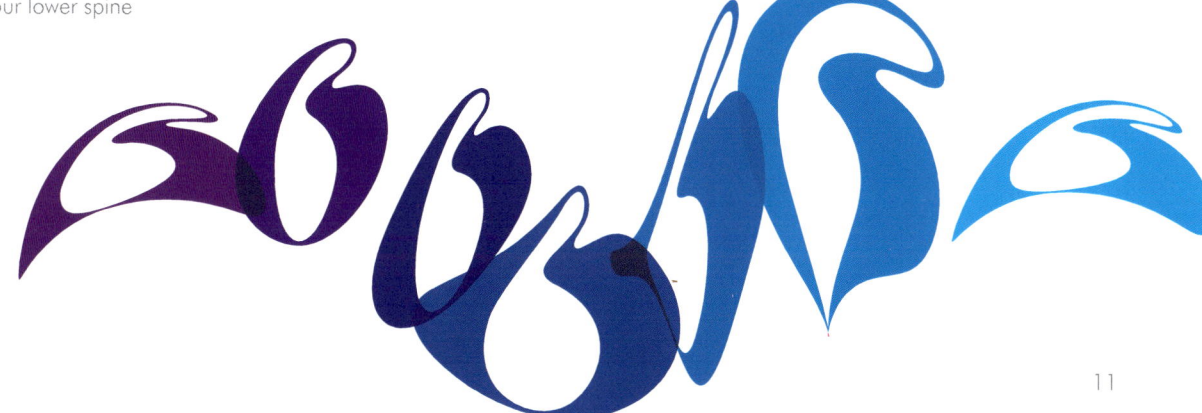

Practice 4: Balancing Breath (Sama Vritti) – When the Components of the Breath are Equal

Effects: Balancing, slightly tonifying, stimulating. Good for low energy, depression, lethargy.

- *Sama* means 'equal' or 'same,' and *vritti* means 'wave' or 'movement.' *Sama Vritti* means that the length or movement of your inhalation and exhalation are equal. Normally, the length of your inhale is shorter than your exhale. But if you consciously make the inhalation and exhalation the same length, you increase the effects of the inhalation as well.

Lengthen both parts of the breath simultaneously. Observe how you feel practicing this ratio. The important thing is the smoothness of your breath. Do this breathing ratio, or a variation of it, to energize, stimulate, and create more focus (see Figure 1).

Practice 5: Reducing and Nourishing Breaths (Visama Vritti) – When the Components of the Breath are Not Equal

In this lesson, the length of your inhalation and exhalation are unequal and can be used to create different effects — either nourishing or reducing your energy.

Classically, the 'nourishing' and 'balancing' breaths are used in the morning or afternoon, and the 'reducing' breath is used in the evening — building in the A.M. and reducing in the P.M. However, let the breathing practice support what's happening in your system now. In other words, you decide what you need, and when you need it. Let your body tell you what practice you need.

'As you lengthen your exhalation, you will create a reducing and relaxing effect in your body and mind'

Figure 1 Lengthening Both Your Inhale And Exhale

Inhalation	HOLD	Exhalation	HOLD	Repeat
8	2	8	2	x4
8	4	8	2	x4
10	4	10	4	x4
10	6	10	6	x4
12	6	12	6	x4
8	0	8	0	x4

Figure 2 Lengthening Your Exhale

Inhalation	HOLD	Exhalation	HOLD	Repeat
8	2	8	2	x4
8	2	10	2	x4
8	2	10	4	x4
8	2	10	6	x4
8	2	12	6	x4
8	0	8	0	x4

The Effects of Reducing Your Breath:

Calming, reducing of agitation, anger, fear, anxiety.

Progressively Lengthen Your Exhalation and Hold (see Figure 2)

You may prepare your body first by moving a little or practicing some yoga postures — placing an emphasis on your exhalation.

As you lengthen your exhalation, you will create a reducing and relaxing effect in your body and mind. Longer holds may bring up strong emotions. And lengthening the exhalation and holding after you exhale can be very challenging. After you exhale, you are empty. There is nothing there, only yourself. Observe how you feel practicing this, and use it as a guide. Modify it in any way you need to.

The Effects of Nourishing Your Breath:

Tonifying, energizing. Builds energy and focus.

Progressively Lengthen Your Inhalation and Hold (see Figure 3)

You may prepare your body first by moving a little, or practicing some yoga postures — placing an emphasis on your inhalation.

Lengthening your inhalation creates a nourishing and stimulating effect in your body and mind. Be aware that you may have a tendency to go beyond what is comfortable for you. Be cautious. *Never push your breath.*

Observe how you feel after following this ratio. Afterward, allow your head and neck to move with your breath to relieve any accumulated tension.

You can also progressively lengthen the hold or retention of your breath on both inhalation and exhalation. Depending on which part of the retention or hold you emphasize (after your exhalation or after your inhalation) you will extend the effects of either the inhalation (nourishing) or exhalation (reducing).

Options

1. Use both the breathing ratios in Figures 2 and 3 as a seated breathing practice, or along with various movements or postures, lengthening your inhalation or exhalation as you move in the postures.

2. Create a practice using a combination of the Nourishing Breath and the Reducing Breath in a sequence. This practice gradually builds and increases energy, then returns to calming, relaxing and cooling.

- Begin by lengthening your inhalation until you reach your comfortable maximum. Your exhalation remains free. Finish, and then rest for a few breaths.

- For your next 10 breaths, sustain your maximum inhalation and allow your exhalation to be equal in duration to your inhalation. Finish, and then rest for a few breaths.

- Now lengthen your exhalation until you reach your comfortable maximum. Your inhalation remains free. Finish, and then allow your breathing to come back to normal.

Figure 3 Lengthening Your Inhale

Inhalation	HOLD	Exhalation	HOLD	Repeat
6	2	12	2	x4
8	2	12	2	x4
10	2	12	2	x4
12	2	12	2	x4
12	4	12	2	x4
8	0	8	0	x4

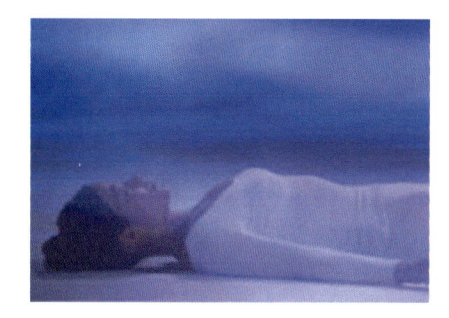

Breathing Rituals: For Body-Mind Recovery

Your Body and Your Breath

Breathing is one of the most important principles of bodily movement, because there is a natural relationship between movement and breath. In yoga, breathing occurs in all poses, from the simplest to the most complex. Every movement is done through a full, conscious breath. Breathing is the best part of the game. So, when you're doing any exercise, whether it's golf or yoga, try to stay deeply aware of your breathing.

Anytime you exercise your body, your movement should be a natural extension of your breath. The action of breathing is what links your attention to your spine's movement. Any movement you make can be observed from your spine's perspective. Reaching for a can of soup on the top shelf extends your spine's muscles. Bending to tie your shoes stretches your lower back. The only difference between this and doing a movement like yoga is that you *consciously intend to move*.

Your spine's health is linked to your whole body's health. Having a youthful, flexible spine means having a youthful, flexible body. Your breathing guides your spine's movement from the inside.

Breathing is the medium through which the movement happens. The postures of yoga, or any intentional movements actually emerge from your breath. As you move, you'll place emphasis on your breathing and how it affects your spine. (See Practice 3 — The Wave.)

**Positive Challenge:
Feel Your Body Now. Breathe More.**
Feeling Your Body This is a simple process that allows you to stay grounded in your body as you breathe. Feeling Your Body is an essential exercise. Come back to it often. It's not complex, and the more you practice it, the simpler it gets, and the deeper it goes.

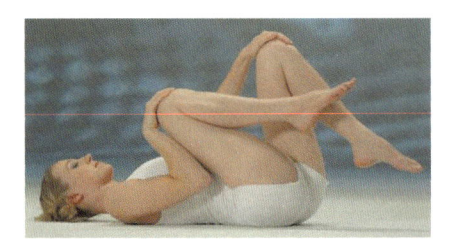

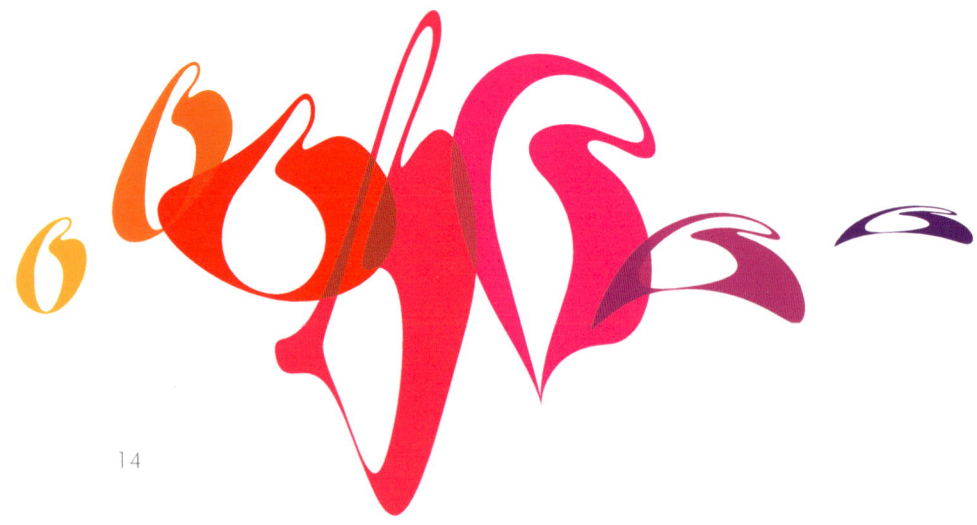

- Find a quiet place to sit down. You may keep your eyes open or closed. Become aware of your natural breathing.

- Observe any sensations you feel. Try not to lose yourself to your thinking mind or to outside distractions. Be fully present in your body and direct your attention to it as much as possible.

- Now, notice where you have your attention at this moment. As you read these words, you're also aware of your surroundings. See if you can be aware of your inner body at the same time. Keep your attention within. Pull it into focus.

- Stay aware of yourself in your body. Let yourself become *aware of your breathing* for a moment and notice any feelings of discomfort in your body. At the same time, notice that the sun is shining, the dog is barking, and the people in the next room are talking. Keep breathing and notice that all this is happening in a remarkable relationship between you, your breathing, and everything you observe. This effortless maneuver is both spontaneous and extraordinary. In this state, there is total acceptance. You're simply observing what's already happening in your natural ordinary awareness.

This experience doesn't need to take long. But spending a few minutes in contact with yourself and your breathing is one of the most important tools of self-inquiry and self-care, leading to balance and self-monitoring. Inevitably, it will become a cornerstone in your self-care and mind-body practice.

'Breathing is one of the most important principles of bodily movement, because there is a natural relationship between movement and breath'

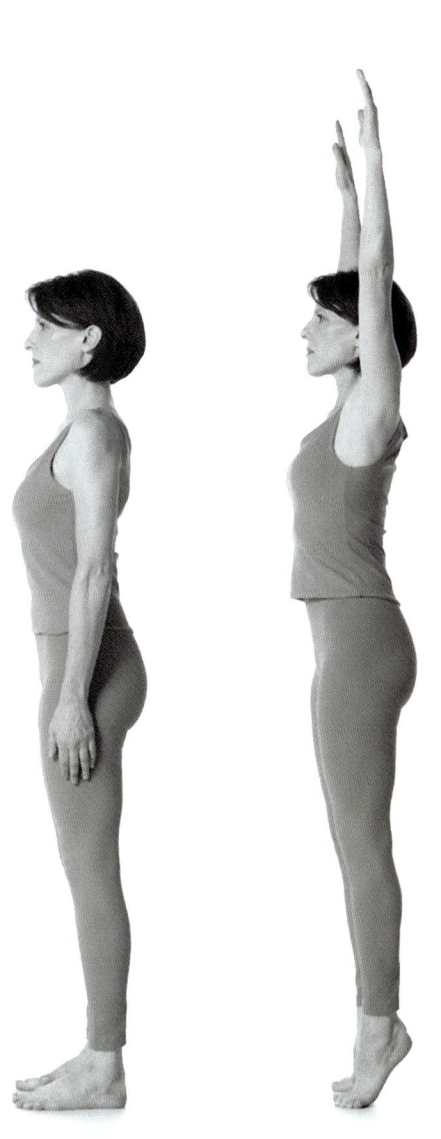

Standing and Moving With Breath

This is a simple movement that will teach you how to move and breathe together in one fluid process. Remember to breathe fully and deeply in this posture. It helps you to keep your attention inward and supports a meditative state. It also engages your muscles, and sends tone, energy, and awareness throughout your body.

Start — Stand with your arms at your sides, lengthen your head and neck, and widen your back.

Inhale — Rise onto your toes, and bring both of your arms overhead.

Exhale — Lower your arms as you come back to standing.

Repeat — 8 times, progressively lengthening your inhalation and the hold after your inhalation — holding 0, 2, 4, then 6 seconds — repeating each (2 times).

Extend your spine and lift your head slightly on inhalation as you lift your arms. Bring your chin slightly down on exhalation as your arms come down.

'Feeling Your Body' is an except from *Emotional Yoga: How the Body Can Heal the Mind* (Simon and Schuster, 2002)

Your Mind and Your Breath

Your mental capacity allows you to focus your attention and engage in many tasks that help you organize your life. When you challenge yourself mentally, it's very important to also create a balance between the energy you expend and recover. Otherwise, when you push yourself beyond your mind's capacity over a long period of time, especially under high-pressure with limited recovery and rest patterns, you end up with burnout, impaired performance, and mental decline.

As a practice, breathing helps you recuperate. Think of breathing as 'down time.' It's a fast and powerful way to manage your mental stress.

Positive Challenge: Be Smarter for Life. Breathe Now.

Check in Breath Instead of checking your email, check in with your breath! Stop. And notice where you are this moment. Are you available to yourself? Can you see where you're not? Jump into present-moment awareness. And notice your breath. Is it short? Is it shallow? Does it gradually get deeper when you stay with it a while longer?

It's amazing how often we're asleep to the power and knowing *of our own presence*. And how even a casual reminder can open our eyes to something entirely different.

Breathing and Sound Meditation

(see Figure 4) This meditation uses your breath, and the repetition of a sound (internally). Use it as a guide to direct your attention away from distractions. Adapt it, and experiment.

- Sit in a comfortable position and breathe 12 times, gradually increasing the length of your exhalations. Then, sit quietly for a moment.

- Repeat the two-syllable sound *Ah – Hum* in your mind, but not out loud. (*Ah-hum* means, 'that which is always there,' 'that which cannot be destroyed.')

- Increase the length of the sound in your mind, using the following lines below (see Figure 4) as a reference. Increase the length of the sound progressively until you get to the longest length of the sound, and then decrease it back to the shortest length. Take your time.

- It's okay if you find yourself breathing as you mentally repeat the sound. You can make this a longer meditation by increasing the number of repetitions.

- You can also use any number of sounds. For example, try: *Ah – Ha – Va*. Or try, *Ra – Ma*, or *Na – Ma*, or *Ah – Men*.

- After you're done, sit quietly for a moment with your eyes closed. Feel the silence inside, and notice the clarity of your attention.

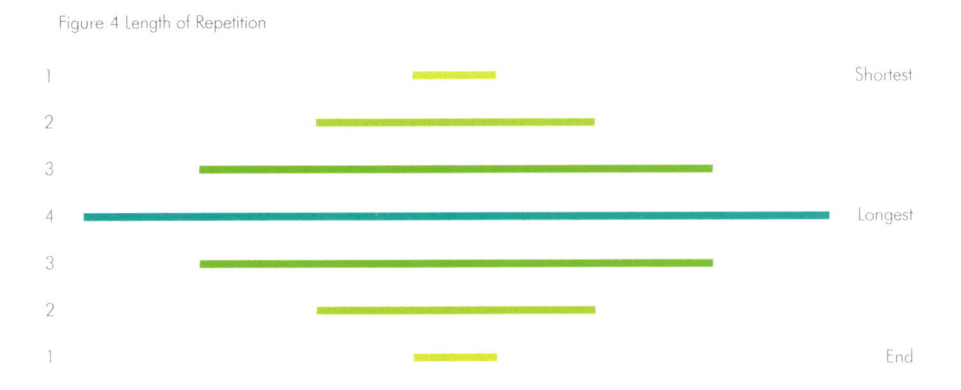

Figure 4 Length of Repetition

'Breathing feels good. It brings emotional sanity'

Your Emotions and Your Breath

Emotions are physical, not psychological. Scientists are beginning to understand this now. Emotions act as a bridge between your body and mind. You are a psychosomatic network, but this doesn't mean that whatever you're experiencing in your body is not to be taken seriously — quite the contrary. Psychosomatic means that your body, mind, and emotions are intimately intertwined.

Emotions and health are intimately connected. Moods and attitudes directly influence your body. Lingering, unresolved, distressing emotions are toxic and a risk factor to your health. But when you're acknowledging, understanding, and expressing emotions, it is as valuable as any healing intervention available. By getting in touch with your emotions, both by listening to them and directing them through your body-mind, you can gain access to the healing wisdom that is your natural and biological right. Make a conscious decision to enter your body-mind's conversation so *you can heal what you can feel*. This is good medicine.

Understanding how your thoughts and your feelings affect every single hormone and cell in your body, and knowing how to change them in a way that is health-enhancing, gives you access to the most powerful and empowering health-creating secret on earth. Breathing is the key to this healing.

'Breathing is good medicine'

Positive Challenge: Feel Better for Life. Breathe More.
Telling Your Emotional Truth
First, sit someplace comfortable. Tune in to your body, focus your attention on your breath, and listen to its flowing rhythm. Put your attention on your heart and ask yourself the following questions. After each one, close your eyes, take a moment, and feel the answer.

- What feeling am I allowing right now?
- What am I not allowing myself to feel?
- Right now, what I am scared to say or feel is…
- What I really want to say or feel is…
- In this situation the real truth is…

Emotional stability is the nexus of a healthy life. Years ago, I investigated the link between yoga and emotional health, which later became my book, *Emotional Yoga: How the Body Can Heal the Mind* (Simon & Schuster, 2002). For more information, go to www.BijaB.com

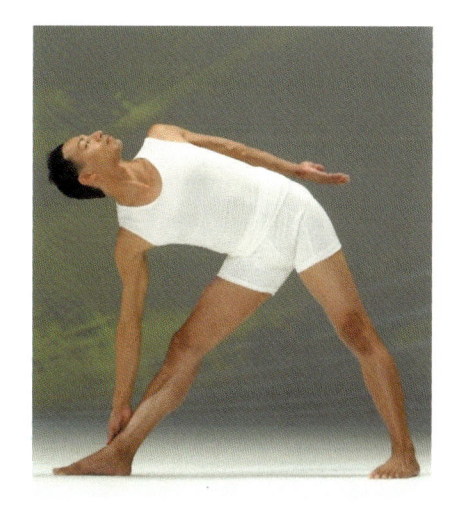

17

Your Immunity and Your Breath

Immunity is a biological term describing a state where the physiology has sufficient defenses to avoid infection, disease, or any other unwanted biological invasion. It's the body's capacity to resist anything harmful it encounters. Strong immunity gives you immediate protection as your body adapts and the immune system prepares itself for future challenges.

Breathing is a way to regenerate your immune system and to build stability, adaptability, and strength. It controls regeneration, which leads to an efficient metabolism. Keep in mind that you are trying to become healthy in all areas of your life. Be consistent and deliberate, and your new habits will motivate you even more as they become linked to a long-term vision of your health.

'Breathing is a powerful way to regenerate your immune system'

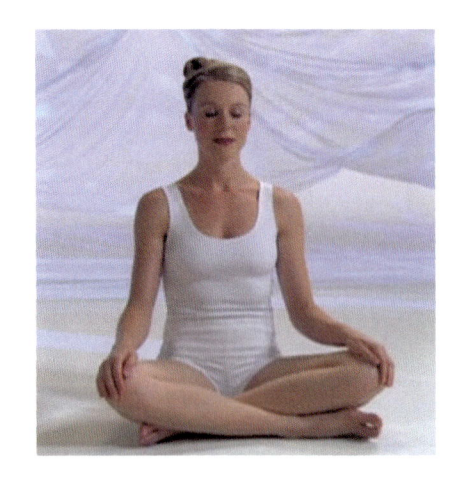

Positive Challenge: Be Healthier for Life. Breathe More.

This practice, an ancient breathing technique that helps you build immunity and strength, involves breathing in stages or steps. I like to think of going up or down in an elevator and stopping at every floor. For example: *Exhale, pause. Exhale, pause. Exhale, pause. Exhale, pause.* Or, *inhale, pause. Inhale, pause. Inhale, pause.* Move with your breath to the bottom floor, or all the way to the top. These have the same effects as lengthening each part of the breath, as in the Nourishing and Reducing Breaths.

Breathing in Stages
Inhalation in Steps Effects:
Nourishing, tonifying, energizing.

As you take in a breath, inhale one-half of your breath comfortably, then pause. Inhale the other half of your breath, then pause.

Exhale completely and fully. Repeat this for 4 breaths. Repeat this again in three stages: inhale one-third, pause; inhale one-third, pause; inhale one-third, pause. Exhale completely. You can continue this pattern four more times or stay with one variation for a total of 8 to 12 breaths.

Be aware of your inhalations, as you emphasize the expansion of the upper chest first, then expand the middle and the lower rib cage. Progressively expand your inhalation from the top down.

Exhalation in Steps Effects:
Reduces agitation; purifying, calming.

Exhale one-half of your breath slowly, pause, then exhale the remaining half of your breath, and pause. Inhale fully. Repeat 4 times. Repeat this again in three stages: exhale one-third, pause; exhale one-third, pause: exhale one-third, and pause. Inhale fully. Repeat 4 more times, continuing this pattern or staying with one variation for a total of 8 to 12 breaths.

Be aware of your exhalations, contracting the abdominal muscles progressively from the pubic bone to your navel, and from your navel to the solar plexus.

Options You may breathe in stages as a seated breathing practice or along with various postures, or *asanas* — moving, then pausing, moving, then pausing, either on your inhale or exhale.

Breathing into Life

Breathing is the expression of life, the pulsation of all that exists. Everything in creation breathes. It's in the movement of the stars, the planets, the earth, the ocean waves, the wind in the trees. These impulses, these frequencies, these rhythms of creation, are expressions of the universal breath of life. This living breath is the same breath that exists within our own bodies.

Breath is the fundamental link between all things in nature. It's our conscious relationship to life. Breathing connects our awareness to every movement, every thought, every emotion we have. How we breathe is how we live. And the way we breathe can allow us to recover our balance of body and mind.

Creating a living balance simply means *restoring our memory of wholeness*, connecting us back to the source of our consciousness. Our breath keeps us in contact with this source, uniting our individual life with all of life.

As we learn to reawaken the natural flow of our breath, we begin to heal ourselves. By using the breath to move our attention within the body, we explore the ever-shifting flow of energy that creates our inner experience. We begin to develop a conscious familiarity with ourselves. We begin to discover the powerful intelligence that's already breathing within us. We begin *Breathing into Life*.

> 'Breathing is one of the greatest secrets of yoga. If you practice it with sincerity, you will obtain healing powers beyond your imagination'

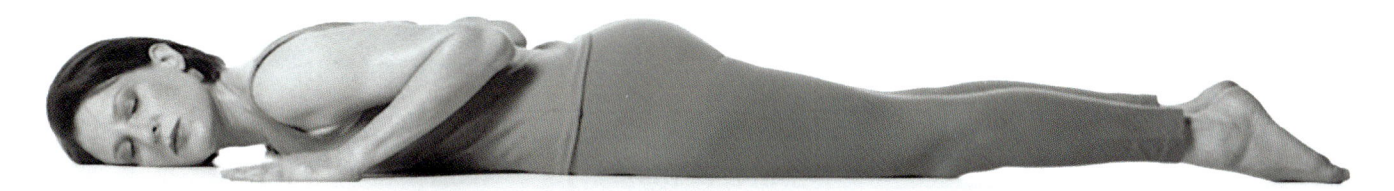

Bija Bennett is a Chicago-based author, artist, and filmmaker who is able to convey the tenets of mind-body health in remarkably engaging ways. Founder of the international lifestyle company, YogaAway LLC, she has produced numerous films on health, yoga, lifestyle, and culture that combine the healing and performing arts. As an entrepreneur and public speaker, she shares her insights with diverse audiences, enabling them to live a healthy, balanced, and meaningful life.

BijaB.com

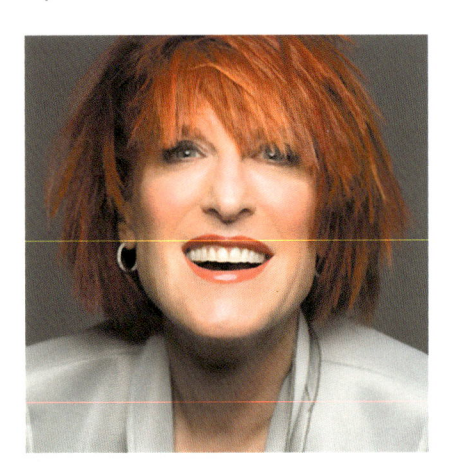

Chicago, Illinois | United States of America
bijab@bijab.com | www.bijab.com

CPSIA information can be obtained at www.ICGtesting.com
Printed in the USA
LVIW01n1138260216
476844LV00008B/50

9 781504 343688